26 Ways to Manage Your Type 2 Diabetes & Control Your Blood Sugar

By

Kimberly Peters

For

26 Ways.com

Other Publications from 26Ways.com:

26 Ways to Save Money on Your Utility Bills

26 Ways to Get More Fun from RC Aircraft

26 Ways to Grow Your On-Line Business

Look for new titles on our website:

http://www.26ways.com

Disclaimer

This is a book designed to give you some helpful insight into how you can control your diabetes and lower your blood sugar. It is NOT designed to be used as a substitute for a Doctor's care or advice. We are not doctors nor do we pretend to be. Everyone is different and everyone's situation is different. We urge everyone with Diabetes to have regular visits with his or her doctor and to follow their guidance and advice above all else. Not everything in this book will pertain to everyone. The writers and publishers of this book assume no responsibility for the application or use of any or all parts of this publication.

Table of Contents

Introduction   5

See Your Doctor(s)   8

Know Your A1c   12

Change a Routine   18

Eat Healthy Meals   23

Eat Consistently   27

Eat More Often   30

Enjoy Healthy Carbs   34

Get Enough Fiber   37

Eat Whole Grains   40

Control Portion Size   42

Eat Healthy Snacks   48

Bring Lunch with You Instead of Dining Out   55

Use Diabetic Energy Bars   57

Make an Appointment   60

Try Cinnamon   63

Create a More Active Lifestyle   65

Lose a Bit of Weight   70

Use a Pedometer or Exercise Band   82

Leave the Car Home!   88

Monitor Blood Pressure   90

Monitor Cholesterol   94

Reduce Stress   96

Check Your Feet   99

See an Eye Doctor   103

Stop Smoking   105

Get Flu Shots   108

Replace Sugary Drinks   111

Vinegar May Reduce Glucose Surge   117

Never Adjust Meds   119

Join a Support Group   123

Brush, Floss, and See a Dentist   125

Get a Full Night's Sleep   127

Stay Away from Steroids   129

Talk to Your Doctor About Supplements   131

Create a Testing Routine   133

Keep a Testing & Food Log   137

Conclusion   140

Introduction

Type 2 Diabetes can be a tough and frightening disease to manage if you do not have a plan or approach. The disease impacts every aspect of your life at some point or another and it is important that you take control of your approach early to limit your chances of some pretty severe side effects.

People with Type 2 Diabetes can live a nice long and productive life if they take the steps necessary to control what they do and how they live their lives. It is not so much how you accomplish your goals but rather how you go about it and for how long.

This book is focused not on specific medical advice but rather common sense things EVERY diabetic should be aware of when it comes to managing the disease. Because you really can't cure it or beat it, but you most certainly can manage it.

Right up front we want to point out that this book, while chocked full of a lot of common sense information, should NOT be used as a substitute for going to see your doctor on a regular basis. EVERY diabetic NEEDS to see their doctors regularly and have regular bloodwork as well. Seeing your doctor at the recommended intervals allows your doctor to discover warning signs early so the effects are minimized.

The other thing we need to point out before we get started is that it is not only important to go and see your doctor, you also have to listen to what they tell you! It will do little good if you go to the doctor and then dismiss their recommendations and advice because you don't think it is all that important!

We should also understand that everyone is different. What works for me might not work for you and vice versa. You might also find that some of the tips or material in this book might not be applicable to you and that's OK. You don't have to do everything in the book to achieve awesome results. Just pick a few things and go with them. Every little thing you do will help you control your blood sugar. It is up to you and what you need to accomplish that will govern what you need to do. So pick and choose and get started!

The last thing we would like to point out is that this disease is controllable. You CAN make a huge impact on your future by taking the appropriate action today!

By taking small steps today to help reduce your blood sugar, you can dramatically decrease the likelihood that you will have serious complications tomorrow. While this is not a guarantee, it is true for a large percentage of diabetic patients.

So with all of this mind, let's start looking at ways we can help control diabetes by lowering blood sugar and increasing our body's ability to deal with the other effect of the disease.

See Your Doctor(s)

About 15 years ago I went to the doctor for a routine yearly physical. IN advance I had completed the standard bloodwork and went to the appointment with the expectation that everything was fine and to come back again in 6 months. After all, I was fairly young and this had been the result of every physical I have had so far in life.

Besides, I had felt fine. No aches, pains, headaches or other problems to worry about or even cause concern. As far as I knew I was the picture of health and there was no indication that this physical was going to be any different. Like I said, I was fairly young and still thought I was invincible.

But the doctor told me that my blood work had come back and that I was a diabetic! Not going to be a diabetic or could be a diabetic but that I WAS a diabetic! I was surprised because I had not had one single symptom. Or so I thought.

Yeah, I was a little thirsty at times but that was about it. So he gave me a prescription for some medication designed to reduce my blood sugar and to have blood work done again in 6 months and come back to see him.

I didn't do much of anything different during those 6 months because, quite frankly, I wasn't exactly sure what I should do in the first place. But I went back in 6 months and the tests once again showed high sugar and it was at that point he referred me to an Endocrinologist.

An Endocrinologist is a doctor who specializes in disease involving the body's endocrine system and diabetes is the most common of those diseases. Now, when you are told to see a specialist, the message sinks in a bit more that this is something to be taken seriously. So off I went to see the new doctor.

The Endocrinologist was a nice fellow who explained to me what was going on and gave me a blood glucose meter and showed me how to test my blood sugar. It was a little scary at first until he showed me and it was nothing. So we went over when to test, how often to test, and when we might want to test more often than other times.

Fortunately for me at the time my "numbers" were still pretty good and I was on the low side or what diabetic levels usually are. Over the years medications were added or changed to address changes in my blood glucose and both my family doctor and the endocrinologist worked together to keep me healthy and on the right track.

I strongly suggest you develop a good relationship with BOTH of your doctors (if you have an Endocrinologist). While your "endo" will address the diabetes aspect of your care, it is your family doctor, or General Practitioner, who will take care of the rest of your health issues and care. While both doctors will help care for you, having them both work together will give you a much better chance of dealing with your diabetes effectively.

Since I see the Endocrinologist 4 times a year and have blood work done each time, I always bring my most current blood work with me to give to my family doctor. This lets him see how I am doing as well. Plus, it sometimes keeps me from having to go for the same bloodwork twice!

Chances are your doctors will also involve others in your care as well. An eye doctor, a foot doctor and a cardiologist might be recommended because of increased risks for certain health problems because of the diabetes. Whatever is suggested you should do. Just because you have no symptoms does not mean you don't have any problems!

I also find that having to go to the doctor routinely gives me an added incentive to watch my weight more closely and also be more aware of my blood sugar levels as well. After all, we want to get good reports so we don't have to take more pills or get "yelled at" by our doctors. Most people want to make their doctors happy and if you are one of them, this can give you an added bonus for seeing your doctors!

Had I not gone to the doctor all those years ago I might have lived with extremely high blood sugar for years and years. All that time the blood sugar would have been damaging my body is several ways all without giving symptoms until severe damage was done! So if you take nothing else from this book, PLEASE, visit your doctors regularly and pay attention to what they tell you.

You will look back years from now and thank yourself for paying such close attention to your health and diabetes now. As we said, you cannot cure diabetes but you sure can manage it. Getting the proper medical team together now will help you both now and later.

Know Your A1c

If you are a diabetic who has been to their doctor than hopefully you are well versed in what an A1c test is and why the results of those tests are so important when it comes to managing your diabetes. Every diabetic should know what their A1c is and how it has been trending over the last several years. This will help you better manage the disease and fend off serious side effects.

The Hemoglobin A1c test is a test that gives an indication of how well you have controlled your blood glucose over the last 3 months. This is important because while we might have a "bad" day or two at times, how well we control over glucose levels over a long period of time is more accurate and informative.

Your best source for information on how to use this test result should come from your health care team. They will provide you with the appropriate levels they would like you to achieve at any given time in your treatment.

For the purpose of this chapter and this book, we will give you a practical lesson on this test and how you can use it to help you manage your diabetes. But again, everyone is different and you should discuss this with your endocrinologist or family doctor for you specific situation.

You are tested for your A1c levels through a simple blood test done at your local lab. The test result will be a number somewhere between 5% and 14% which will be a whole number plus tenths. So your result might be 5.6 or 7.8 or thereabouts.

Generally speaking the levels for non-diabetics will be 4 or low fives. Generally speaking, your A1c should be below 7.0 with some doctors liking it to be 6.5 or below depending on your own health condition and situation.

It is important for EVERY diabetic patient to know his or her A1c levels because it lets them know how much they need to do or change in order to get down to a safe or desired level.

For example, if your A1c test comes back at 6.1%, then you are doing quite well and will probably just have to maintain what you are now doing or just make some minor changes. But if your A1c came back at 9% then your doctor will likely take some significant steps in changing medication or your treatment plan.

But knowing your A1c is important for another reason as well and that is for trending. Trending is how well you are doing over longer periods of time such as 1,2,3 or more years. For example, if you are seeing your A1c climbing slightly with every test, then you might wish to take more proactive actions because what you are currently doing is becoming gradually less effective.

But if your reading before your last test was 6.5 and your last test was 7.0 and your current test was 6.4 then perhaps you had something going on during that one test that caused a temporary spike such as a sickness or infection.

Spikes are one thing but a constant increase over long period of time is something else.

Conversely, you are seeing a steady lowering of your A1c then that is great because what you are doing is still as effective as it had been so your efforts are really paying off for you. This will keep you encouraged and motivated to keep on doing what you are doing.

Knowing your A1c is an important tool in understanding how well you have your blood glucose controlled over extended periods of time. It is a more accurate reflection than individual blood glucose tests that give you results of what your glucose is at that particular instant.

The A1c test generally consists of a 90 day time frame and half of the result comes from the first 45 days or so and the other half from the last 45 days. So if you know you had high glucose levels for a while due to a health issue or sickness, that would impact have the result of the test. Though the results would still be higher, at least you would know why they might be a bit higher than usual.

The A1c test is just part of the overall blood work that you will have a few times a year if you are a diabetic. The purpose is to not make you feel bad or scare you but instead to provide you with an indication of how your body is responding to your efforts to control your sugars. Minor daily spikes which might cause alarm during a daily test will not play that large a role in an A1C test (unless there are a LOT of those spikes) and the overall result will be more accurate.

If you have had blood work done but do not know what your A1C is, then ask your doctor because it is important that you know. I always ask for a copy of my test results and I save all of them in a folder so I can look back to see if there are any trends that I need to be aware of. Though your doctor should be doing this as well, remember you are one of many patients your doctor cares for. But you are the only patient that YOU have to be concerned about.

Do not accept your doctor's statement that your tests came back "normal". Norma is a relative term and you should know what is normal for you.

Get a copy of the bloodwork and if you have any questions or concerns, ask your doctor to explain them. Once you understand what each result means and what it refers to, you will have a much better grasp on what you need to do in order to live a healthier lifestyle.

Another reason to have copies of your tests might be if you were to switch doctors or go to see a specialist for some reason. You will then have a history of blood work to share with the new doctor so they can make better and more informed decisions.

Change a Routine

Before we get into what we have to do, let's talk for a minute about how we can successfully change something we are doing so we have lasting results with far less of a chance of falling back into our "old" ways.

Whenever we have to change something that has become a habit, we need to identify the behavior we need to change and substitute another behavior that will help us get better or different results. It is not enough to simply stop doing something. We need to substitute a good behavior for the bad behavior.

When we try to stop doing something bad, let's say eating an ice cream sundae every night that spikes our glucose levels, and don't substitute something else in its place, we have to rely on something most people call "willpower".

The problem is that willpower for most of us is a myth. For most of us, changing something we do by forcing ourselves to do it is at best a temporary solution. Because over time, we will lose the ability to stick to that behavior and we will backslide and eventually go back to what we had been doing or worse.

Think about the people who want to lose weight and go on a strict diet where they eat nothing but vegetables and water. Granted, if they eat just a vegetables and drink a ton of water they will lose weight. But the problem is that few people can, or should, stick to that diet for the rest of their lives.

So they lose 10 pounds, start "cheating" by eating just a little of what they really like and then they eat more and more of it until they gained back all the weight they lost plus they gained an additional 5 pounds! This kind of "yo-yo dieting" is the most common side effect of diets and it occurs primarily because we cannot change something long-term by forcing ourselves to sacrifice.

The best chances of results occur when we lessen the sacrifice and make changes that we find easy but are still effective.

For example, if we stop eating that sundae and substitute something else that we enjoy that is low in carbs or sugars, the net effect will be a positive one as far as blood glucose is concerned.

Plus, we are not sacrificing or burdening ourselves in the process. We won't have the hunger pangs and temptations that come from an empty stomach and a weakened mind.

The other aspect of change that is important is the need to make whatever changes we need to make manageable. Sometimes this can be difficult if the situation is urgent but most of the time we have some time in which to make those changes.

For example, let's say your A1c is 8.9 and your doctors want to see it under 7. That is a significant drop and it might be better, if your doctor agrees, to set a goal to drop it to 7.9 in 3 months and then to under 7 in 6 months. This will give you a chance to make changes in stages instead of all at once. Sometimes this is not possible but most of the time it is.

The point is that sometimes really aggressive goals might seem overwhelming or impossible to achieve.

It's like the person who is told they need to lose 100 pounds. A 100 pound weight loss goal might intimidate the heck out of someone. But if they were told to try and lose 2 pounds a week, that doesn't seem all that difficult and more people would at least try to sustain their efforts.

Smaller goals also tend to show more positive reinforcement and progress than large goals as well. It is much easier to pat yourself on the back at the end of the week when you lost those two pounds than it is when you have lost 4 pounds and tell yourself "4 down 96 to go!"

When it comes to diabetes, there are several routines that you either need to modify or start. All of these will be discussed in this book and perhaps some additional ones will be suggested by your medical team. But whatever you need to do, do it in such a way that you will have the best possible chance for long-term success.

To start, try and few a few easy and simple things to either change, start or stop. This will help get you in the right frame of mind and help get you motivated by seeing how your efforts are bringing your blood sugar down.

Then, as those things become habits and you do them almost without thinking, add something else into the mix to get even better results.

Do not try and do too much too soon. Work with your medical team to come up with a plan that you think will work for you. Be honest with your doctors and with yourself when it comes time to telling what you think you are capable of doing. It is not about getting massive results in the very beginning. (Unless this is necessary due to your particular situation. Check with your medical team and follow their guidance.)

Remember it is much better to do something smaller for a long period of time than to try and do too much only to give up when the effort becomes too great.

Slow and steady winds the race!

Eat Healthy Meals

So much of our overall health comes from what we put in our bodies. The food we eat and the liquids we drink play a crucial role in how our bodies grow, how our immune systems function and how we handle the day to day stresses of normal life.

Diabetes is a disease that forces us to be more knowledgeable about the foods we eat, how much of them we eat, when we eat them and how our bodies react to them. If we do not approach eating with all of these factors in mind, we will not get the optimum results we need as far as tight glucose control.

I urge everyone to go out and purchase a diabetes cookbook and a book that lists the carbs and glycemic index of all common foods.

This will help you not only plan meals better, but get better results with less effort and sacrifice. Sometimes just substituting one food for a close equivalent can make a huge difference. But you will never know unless you have some way of finding this information out.

Many people believe that diabetics can't have anything sweet or rich and that is just not the case. You can still have those things you just have to structure your eating habits to include a LITTLE bit of those things along with healthy foods and vegetables.

For example, if you love chocolate, maybe you can have a small piece every now and then without raising your blood sugar. The key sometimes is just portion size. Have one small piece instead of the entire one pound bar! Talk to your doctor to see what you can and can't have.

Meals should be lower in carbohydrates but not carbohydrate free! Everyone needs a certain level of carbohydrates in their diet but it depends on where you get them from. You can get carbs from grains or mashed potatoes and you can get them from hot fudge and sugary drinks.

So your choice is not carb-free but healthy versus unhealthy carbs.

You also have to watch out for certain dietary approaches and recommendations for people who are not diabetics. For example, have a wide array of colors of food on your plate usually refers to fruits and vegetables on your dinner or lunch plate. But a diabetic can have a plate full of brightly colored fruits and have a whopping amount of carbs on their plate because certain fruits are loaded with sugar and carbs! So make sure whatever approach you take it is one approved for diabetics and focused on carb control.

The best source for dietary guidelines will be your medical team. Most health insurance plans will cover the cost of a dietician consultation or program for diabetics. Check with your plan. If your plan offers a free consultation, take advantage of it.

The dietician will help design a plan for you based on the foods that you like to eat. It is not about eating foods you hate or tasteless foods you have to drown in sauces or wash down with water.

It is all about coming up with a plan that you can embrace and stick to that will allow you to have tasty and delicious meals that are still responsible at the same time.

Eat Consistently –

Do Not Skip Meals (especially breakfast!)

Sometimes our schedules do not permit us to eat like we really want to. So we either skip meals entirely as we rush out the door to catch a bus or train or we scarf down a carb loaded bagel or buttered roll from the cafeteria for breakfast. Neither is a great choice.

Skipping meals, especially breakfast, is not a good thing at all for anyone but especially for diabetics. Skipping meals can result in wild swings of blood glucose as our bodies are alternately starved and binged over the course of the day.

When we skip a meal, our blood sugar drops because we are not introducing any food into our system. But when the sugar drops, our insulin levels change as well so we do not have a low sugar reaction. But when we have our next meal, our insulin levels are not prepared for the new food and our blood sugar skyrockets because there is not the right amount of insulin in our blood to handle the carbs we just ingested.

We are much better off when we establish a set schedule for when and how we eat. This allows our body to "learn" our eating schedule and adapt itself to what it knows should be coming into our bodies after meals. This doesn't mean eating the same thing every day but it means eating a pretty much the same time every day and eating roughly the same amount of carbs at a meal.

Our goals should not be to have our glucose levels really low for part of the day and really high for other parts of the day. Instead our goals should be to have fairly stable glucose levels throughout the day without the wild highs or lows.

While our glucose levels will go higher after meals we want to keep those spikes fairly reasonable. The usual guideline is to have glucose levels of 180 or less 2 hours after a meal. Your medical team might have other guidelines or targets for you based on your own situation and condition.

Skipping meals also makes you lose energy and greatly increases the desire to snack throughout the day. Since snack foods are usually not the healthiest food options for diabetics we want to keep the urges to binge and snack to a minimum. We should plan on getting the bulk of our nutrition from the foods we eat during our regularly scheduled meals and not through snacking or bingeing. A snack every once in a while is usually OK, but we should not make it a habit. When we do snack, make it a healthy and low carb snack such as a protein or energy bar or a diabetic nutrition bar, Stay away from fatty foods like chips or sugary food like candy, pastries or ice bream.

Eat More Often

Here is a suggestion that might seem counter intuitive but could also work wonders for you in stabilizing your glucose levels. Instead of eating three full sized meals throughout the day, eat more often but consume less at each meal.

The idea behind this is to allow your body to keep its insulin levels at the same level throughout the day but consuming your foods more often so they are introduced into the body more frequently but in fewer quantities. This means spreading your calories and carbs over more meals throughout the day.

That does not mean we get to eat more often and eat the same amount as we used to eat!

What it means is that if your daily calorie intake was 2,000 over three meals, eating more often would take those same 2,000 calories and spread them out over 5 meals. So instead of consuming 666 calories per meal you would be consuming 400 calories a meal. Sorry to burst your bubble but this works.

The same approach goes for carb control as well. If you have a limit of 150 grams of carbohydrate for the day that would be 50 per meal for 3 meals a day and 30 per meal for 5 meals a day. You do NOT get to eat the same amount of carbs in every meal when you increase the number of meals you have each day! This will defeat the purpose of getting rid of the large highs and lows in your body.

You can also have three primary meals during the day that are slightly reduced and then add a mid-morning and mid-afternoon snack in the mix to help keep your glucose more stable. So find whatever works best for you and then stick to it.

When you eat a meal, your blood sugar might be 90-100 before the meal and 2 hours after the meal.

Then it slowly goes down as your body processes the food. Then the next meal rolls around and it starts all over again from 100 to 180 and back down again. It is like a roller coaster going up and down all day long.

But if we eat less at each meal but eat more often, maybe our pre-meal is 110 and after the meal it only goes up to 140 or 150 and then the cycle repeats over and over again with each meal. The swings which used to be 80 points or more have been reduced to 30-40 points and the result is a more stable blood sugar level throughout the day.

This helps the body avoid having to produce a lot off insulin and then no insulin followed by a lot of insulin over and over all day long. Another benefit is that if you are prone to low sugar episodes, eating more often should help you with that as well. That is because there is more food being processed in your digestive system all day long.

If your lifestyle and schedule allows you to eat smaller meals more often, why not give it a try? It just might be one easy (and sometimes more enjoyable) change that you will have absolutely no problem with!

Just be careful that more meals does not lead to more calories or more carbs!

Enjoy Healthy Carbs

Controlling diabetes is not all about eliminating carbs from your diet. Our bodies need carbohydrates in order to function properly and provide us with the energy we need to make it through the day. So our goal should not be to eliminate carbs but to eat "good carbs" that won't make our glucose shoot into the stratosphere when we eat them.

Carbs also make your sugars rise faster than fats so if you have a lot of carbs in your diet then that will make your sugars higher after your meals. That is why it is so important to limit carb intake and to make the carbs you do eat of the "good" variety.

Though there are exceptions to every rule, when it comes to carbs whole grain carb such as whole wheat flour and brown rice are much better for you than white flour and processed grains such as white rice.

So some good choices for you might be some foods made with whole grain flours, brown rice, cereal made with whole grain ingredients and that also have very little added sugar, whole grain breads, baked potato and even some baked steak fries might give your meals a bit of a tastier appeal.

On the other side of the spectrum, some foods you should always try to avoid or at least limit might be anything made with white flour, white rice, cereals with a lot of added sugar and processed grains, white bread and French fries.

Ask your doctor or nutritionist for a listing of good carbs and bad carbs. Or, go to the library or book store and pick up a book that outlines good dietary choices that also has a chapter on carbs and choose your carbs carefully. Carbs from the "bad" side can be eaten in very limited quantities every once in a while but should not be included in your everyday diet.

Carbs from the "good side" should be part of your everyday diet but you should still monitor your overall consumption of carbs to make sure it still is within your daily limit. As far as "bad carbs" are concerned you can still eat them in very small amounts but they should be reserved for special occasions or rare indulgences.

If you are unsure of what roles and amounts carbs should have in your diet, I suggest you consult with your doctor or nutritionist so you can design an overall diet that will limit total carbs, restrict "bad" carbs and still give your body everything it needs to live a healthy lifestyle. A little planning can go a long way in getting that blood sugar under control and down near normal levels.

Get Enough Fiber

Many diabetics are not aware that fiber is a type of carbohydrate. But fiber is also a carbohydrate that is not broken down by the body which also means that fiber does not raise glucose levels in the body. But fiber also does a few other things in the body that are good for diabetics.

There are two types of fiber. Soluble fiber and insoluble fiber. Insoluble fiber helps keep you digestive tract operating smoothly and properly. This helps you have normal bowel movements and reduces the chance of constipation or diarrhea. Whole wheat bran is a type of insoluble fiber. Soluble fiber, if eaten in large enough amounts, can help lower cholesterol and improve blood glucose control. Oatmeal is an example of soluble fiber.

Fiber also helps you eat less because fiber makes you feel full sooner after you eat foods that contain fiber. So you will tend to eat less with a fiber rich diet and this helps you ingest fewer carbohydrates and that means less spiking of glucose levels after meals.

As with anything in life, when it comes to fiber, you should not eat everything in the supermarket that contains fiber just because it is good for you. Most fiber rich foods also contain other kinds of carbohydrates which are consumed in the human body and that do impact your blood glucose levels.

So choose foods that have high amounts of fiber as well as other carbohydrates and make them part of your overall healthy diet. Most humans should have roughly 20-35 grams of fiber a day and the truth is that most people eat less than that in their everyday diet. Diabetics might want to eat more than that amount because more fiber will make you feel full faster and you will eat less. Check with your doctor or nutritionist about how much fiber you should have in your diet.

Foods that have significant fiber in them are oats, barley, whole-grain breads, fruits, brown rice, nuts, and beans. Foods to stay away from would be processed foods and refined foods. These have little fiber and usually are loaded with calories and "bad carbs". So instead of fast food as a meal, have some oatmeal and fruit. You will feel better, your glucose will be lower, and your gastrointestinal system will operate much better at the same time.

If your diet is low in fiber, add additional fiber slowly so your body gets used to the additional fiber. Otherwise you might find yourself with digestive problems such as constipation. It is also important to drink 6-8 glasses of water every day so that your body always has enough water. This will help you avoid constipation as well.

Eat Whole Grains

Whole grains are not only a great source of fiber but they also are a great source of vitamins and minerals as well. So it just makes sense to make them a part of your overall diet. The ability to have tighter control of your blood glucose levels is another added bonus.

Grains all contain carbohydrates and if you are going to eat them, you might as well choose the grains that will give your body better nutrition and raise your blood sugars less. That means choosing whole grain foods and leaving the processed foods loaded with sugar out of your shopping cart.

Whole grain food use the whole grain of wheat while refined grains such as white flour products use only the starchy parts of the grain which are also the parts that raise our glucose levels! Refined grains also lose much of their nutrients during the refining process so you are eating more "empty" calories.

Reading nutrition labels is an important part of the food selection process. Just because a product features the words "whole grain product" on the front of the package does not mean there is a significant amount of whole grain in the actual food. It might have some whole grains but a very small amount. They advertise whole grains to make the item appear more nutritious and healthier than it really is.

Some examples of whole grain foods are popcorn, brown rice, whole rye, sorghum, buckwheat, whole oats, whole grain corn meal and whole grain barley. Always check the labels on any food before you purchase it to make sure it is not high in bad carbs but also has whole grains in it as well. It is something that might allow you to change your meals and make them tastier and healthier at the same time without sacrificing a thing!

Control Portion Size

Are you aware that your eyes can have a direct impact on glucose control, weight gain or loss, and your overall sense of well-being? Well, they do play an important role when it comes to what we eat and how much we eat. One of the ways our eyes can help us or hurt us is when it comes to portion size.

Portion size is a critical element of any diet. Even the healthiest of foods will cause us to gain weight rapidly if we eat too much of them. Contrary to what most people think, you can have out of control weight gain and blood sugar levels even though you are eating "approved" foods. This happens when we overeat and have huge portion sizes.

Portion size, often referred to as a "serving" is important because portion size has a direct correlation between the number of carbs and calories contained by that food. For example, a healthy whole grain cereal might have only 5 grams of carbohydrates in a single service but if you eat the whole damned box you might end up consuming 70-100 grams of carbohydrates and 2,000 calories all in just one meal!

Portion size is where it really becomes difficult to eat out as well. Today many restaurants subscribe to the "more is better" motto and you get a plate of food that could feed twelve or a burger you could eat for your next 3 dinners! I really believe the world would be a better place, and people far happier and healthier, if restaurants would cut the portion sizes down to normal levels and reduce the prices accordingly. But since that is not likely to happen any time soon, let's see how we can monitor and adjust portion sizes.

One of the most effective ways to control portion size is to place an appropriate amount of food on your plate and just bring that to the table instead of having a huge serving dish or plate on the table.

This way when you are done with what's on your plate you just stop eating. Your eyes won't see the huge platter of roast beef or pasta sitting there just begging to be eaten.

Another effective tool is to use smaller plates. This will help control portion size in two ways. First, a smaller plate will hold less food so there might be an "automatic" reduction in the food you can bring to the table at one time. So as long as you don't use more than one smaller plate, you should be eating less by just reducing plate size.

The other things that smaller plates do is make less food look like more food. You can take the same amount of food and place it on a large plate and a small plate and it will look like more food on the smaller plate because it will cover more of the plate and will probably be stacked or piled a little higher as well.

So your eyes play tricks on you and fool you into thinking you are eating more than you really are!

But regardless of what size plates you are using, you MUST be aware of how much food you are putting on that plate! Even a smaller dish loaded with jelly beans is going to have a ton of sugar and carbs in it. Use measuring cups or other ways of determining the correct portion size and then place that on your plate and no more.

You can also spread your food over a larger area to make it look like more as well. So instead of piling it high on the plate, spread it around and pile it lower. This will make the plate appear to be more full and have more food on it. This is your eyes at work again!

Regardless of the size plates you use, it makes sense to use actual measuring tools to determine the correct portion sizes. If you try and do it by eye then a service could turn into 1.5 servings or 2 or more. Even a little bit more at each meal can have a considerable impact on your sugars and calorie intake at the end of the week. So get some measuring cups and spoons and eat real sized portions!

When you eat out, portion size can become more difficult to control. The restaurant has its own portion size and that is what you are going to get no matter if you eat it, take it home, or throw it out. But there are a few things you might be able to do when it comes to eating out and portion size.

The first thing you can do is ask if they have a reduced portion size option. They might be accommodating to you and offer you less food for a reduced price. I wouldn't count on it but you can ask.

An alternative might be to ask if you could order from the children's menu. Those are smaller versions of their regular entrée's. So instead of having that 12 pound hamburger for $15.00 you might be able to get a quarter pound burger for $5.99. You save carbs, calories and money all at the same time.

You also could share a single entrée with someone else. Just order the entrée and ask for two plates. There might be a small fee to share but you will still overall pay less and you will not over eat.

Another option is to order your entrée and when you order it ask for a container to bring some of it home. Then, instead of eating and taking home what is left over, take the excess food off your plate before you start eating and place it in the container. This will prevent you from gradually picking at what is left and eventually eating most, if not all, of the food right then and there!

It is not always a case where we have to stop eating the foods we love. Sometimes all that is needed to achieve the results we want or need is to eat reasonable sized portions so we do not overload our systems or cause us to gain weight.

Eat Healthy Snacks

For most diabetics, we struggle through the day trying to balance the need to keep our blood sugars level with the need to find healthy foods for meals and snacks. For most of us, meals are easier because we can plan for them and we prepare the majority of them in our own kitchens at home.

Snacks are a different matter at times because while most of us snack at home, some of our snacks occur at work or on the go or while we are out of the house. These are the times when healthy snacks can be difficult or impossible to find.

For example, if you go to the movies, try and find a healthy snack among all the candy, sugary drinks, ice cream bars, hot dogs and nachos!

And even popcorn, one of the healthiest snacks around when we have it at home, is a disaster when you have it at the ballpark or at the movie theatre!

The last time I was at a ball park, a bucket of popcorn, which costs like $322 had over 2,500 calories!!! That is more than you are supposed to consume in an entire day! It's not the popcorn itself that is the problem it is the button and all the salt they put on it that makes it taste so good along with the oil they pop it in that adds all those calories!

Even walking through the mall becomes a challenge when it comes to snack time. Most of the foods people crave and look to purchase are loaded with calories and carbohydrates. Which also means those are the same foods we diabetics should be staying away from.

When it comes to snacks at home I prefer popcorn and fruit. Popcorn is great because it actually is good for you if it is not loaded down with butter and salt. It is also very filling which helps you lose the empty feeling fasting while consuming fewer calories.

Microwave popcorn, which is not as good for you as air-popped popcorn has the advantage of being tasty and easy to prepare with very little mess and cleanup to worry about. You can also get the little "100 calorie" bags that give you enough to satisfy a craving but not enough calories or carbs to cause problems. But if you can air pop your popcorn that is the healthiest way because it uses no oil which means fewer calories. I add a TINY bit of salt for flavor and I'm good to go!

Fruits such as apples are good choices as well because they are filling and take some time to eat meaning you get your calories more slowly than scarfing down 5 Oreos in 2 minutes! Just be careful when it comes to fruit because fruit has natural sugars and carbs in it that can cause blood sugar spikes if you eat too much.

Vegetable type snacks like carrot or celery sticks are great because they are low fat, low calorie and low carb snacks that taste good and fill your up with little to no effect on your blood sugar levels! You can cut up a bunch and place them in a Zip-lock bag with a little water to keep them moist and they will be ready when you need them!

Or, in the case of carrots, buy the bag of baby carrots which are already snack sized!

One thing we really need to watch out for when it comes to snacks are the beverages we use to "wash" those snacks down. Most sodas have a ton of sugars in them which will spike glucose levels sharply. Plus, they are loaded with calories as well. Even fruit juices are sometimes loaded with sugars and carbs.

The best beverage for diabetics and everyone else is good old fashioned water! Water has essential nutrients in it and it hydrates the body very well. Sodas and other drinks sometimes contain salt or sodium which DEHYDRATES the body and this can actually be worse than no water at all!

If you are home, have some water near you at all times. Drinking more water will keep you hydrated as well as giving you a full feeling after drinking it. That can actually reduce the food cravings you get from an empty stomach. Sip it throughout the day instead of drinking too much all at one time.

If you cannot drink water, diet sodas or seltzer are good alternatives if consumed in moderation. But even diet sodas have artificial sweeteners which can make the body crave sugars and also raise your glucose levels. Plus these beverage can have salt which makes you even thirstier later! Do yourself a favor and go with water.

As far as snacks on the go are concerned, I like the exercise bars or diabetic bars that provide high energy snacks to low carb levels. These power bars are small enough to fit in your jacket pocket or purse so you can take them with you wherever you go. When everyone else in the group goes for that huge pretzel with the gallon size soda you can drink an ice cold water and eat a power bar.

But let's say you don't want to go that route and you want to fit in with everyone else. Or, you don't like or have a power bar or similar item with you. In that case, you simply have to make the best choices from whatever is available. For help with that, we need to read nutritional labels.

Depending on where you live, many food stands or locations will post calorie and carbohydrate information on the menu boards or at least have a handout that lists this information on it. If they don't have it posted, you can always go online with your smartphone and do a search for the product in question. Then you can make an informed decision.

This is important because sometimes the oddest choices might make the most sense. For example, based on the calorie information at the ballpark, someone who is on a diet would be much better off calorie wise with the cotton candy over a pretzel or popcorn!!! The cotton candy was 300 calories while the pretzel was 800 calories and the popcorn 1,100 for the small size. Now the cotton candy is nutritionally by far the worst but calorie wise, it was the winner!

I am not recommending anyone eat cotton candy but the example shows us just how important nutrition labels can be when it comes to picking the right snacks. If we need something but there are now healthy snacks available, then we can at least pick the best of the worst as our snack!

The same goes for shopping as well. Look at the labels for the type of snack you want and choose the best option. Sometimes one brand might have far lower carbohydrates than the others. By knowing this you can choose the best items and enjoy your food with far less guilt.

Snacks are good for us when it comes to stabilizing our glucose levels but only if those snacks do not contribute to our eating far more carbs than we are supposed to.

Bring Lunch with You Instead of Dining Out

For reasons that we have already touched on, diabetics have a much tougher time managing their glucose levels when they have to eat out all the time. When our food is prepared by others, we lose the control over what actually goes into that food and the effects it will have on our blood sugars.

When we prepare our own meals, we often study each individual component of that meal and make healthy decisions based on certain information. Something simple as a turkey sandwich can have significant differences between being made at home and one ordered out.

We might buy the bread that has the fewest carbs or the most whole grains. We might choose the turkey with the lowest sodium or salt content. We might use low-fat mayo or other healthier condiments. Last, but certain not least, we can carefully control how much meat, and other ingredients that are put on that sandwich.

When we bring our own lunch with us instead of buying lunch out we get certain benefits. We can control portion size, we control the ingredients and we almost always save money when we make it ourselves. Healthier food choices in restaurants are almost always more expensive and even then we have to take someone else's word that these are really "healthy" alternatives.

Controlling our blood glucose means having control over what goes into the food we consume on a daily basis. When we control more of the overall process we almost always get better results. So bring in instead of ordering out. You'll be healthier, richer, and happier all at the same time.

Use Diabetic Energy Bars or Shakes Instead of a Meal

Another way to limit our intake of carbs without skipping meals is to use a low carb or diabetic milkshake or energy bar in pace of a meal. This enables our body to get the nutrition it needs without consuming high sugar or high fat ingredients.

There are several healthy meal substitutes for diabetics available in supermarkets and health food stores that we can use to substitute for a meal when we are rushed or on the go. It is much better to grab a shake than go through the drive through for a burger and fries.

If you decide to go this route every once in a while, there are a few things you should be aware of when it comes to overall nutrition.

First of all, if you grab a shake or an energy bar in place of a meal, make sure you are getting all the nutrition you need in the other meals you eat that day. The nutrition should be balanced as well. Do not skip breakfast and lunch and substitute shakes instead and then have a monster dinner to get everything else you need for the day. This will place a huge burden on your body to absorb all those carbs and other foods all at one time.

Second, make sure what you are eating IS really a healthy and nutritious products and not some sugary caffeinated so called energy drink. Just because it says healthy on the label doesn't mean it really is. Check the label for ingredients and total carbs and sugars. Pick the best product that suits your tastes.

Third, this should not be something you do every day of the week. Whenever possible, try to have well balanced meals and snacks and stay away from processed products and foods.

These products are good for occasional use when circumstances make sense but not for everyday use.

When you start using these shakes or bars, test your blood sugar two hours after you eat them to see what effect they are having on your body. Everyone is different and if you find your sugars are higher than you expected, try a different product. Test yourself like that after ingesting these products a few times until you get a better idea how your body is reacting to them.

Depending on your own situation and medications, not eating enough at a meal can lead to low blood sugar and that is not good either. If you eat a bar or drink a shake and you find your sugars are getting too low, you might have to add something else to the meal to get your sugars up a bit higher. Adding a few carbs from a piece of bread or a piece of fruit might be all that is needed. But you will only know this if you test yourself a few times to see how your body reacts.

Make an Appointment

with a Dietician

If you insurance company will pay you for a consultation with a nutritionist, or even pay you to attend classes on nutrition, do yourself a favor and take advantage of that. You would be shocked to see how much a few small changes can do for your blood sugar control without impacting your enjoyment of eating.

Controlling sugar levels is just not all about cutting carbohydrate intake. It is all about maintaining a healthy lifestyle, getting to and maintaining a healthy weight, and getting the body everything it needs to help it function normally and fight infection and disease.

That's an awful lot for people like you and I to handle all by ourselves. That's where the nutritionist comes in. They look at where we are and where we need to get to and they give us a healthy and responsible way to get there. Because when it comes to managing diabetes, how we get there is almost as important just getting there.

The nutritionist will give you a personalized meal plan based on your weight, diabetic condition and overall health. That meal plan will have a specific calorie intake and amount of carbohydrates that you can ingest every day. This will help you achieve both nutrition and weight loss goals.

Then, once the amounts have been determined they will work with you to choose foods and meals that fit your tastes. This is not about how much you have to sacrifice but instead how best to create healthy meals that you will truly enjoy.

Many people do much better when they have a plan they just have to follow. If they know what they have to do and have it all laid out for them, they will just follow it.

The trouble comes when they know what they have to do but have no idea how to go about even getting started.

Nutritionists will also explain to you the foods that will have the greatest impact on your blood sugars and which ones will the least impact. Sugars in soft drinks, for example, get right into your blood stream much fast than sugars from other foods. By limiting the sugars and carbs that are rapidly sent into your blood stream and replacing them with slower acting ones, we can dramatically lower spikes that can cause problems.

Proper nutrition is not just important for diabetics but for everyone whether they have any health issues or not. Proper nutrition helps people with health problems deal with them more effectively while also helping to protect them against developing additional problems later on in life.

For diabetics, proper nutrition is one tool we can use to get our A1c down, have fewer glucose spikes, and help shield us from developing significant diabetes related problems in the future.

Try Cinnamon &

Some Gum

Here are two "quick hitters" that might help you for two different reasons:

There have been reports that adding cinnamon to your diet can help lower blood sugar. Not exactly sure if that is true or not because there are many reports that say it does and some that say it doesn't! But cinnamon does make certain foods taste better and will not have a negative effect on blood sugar so you might wish to try it.

Cinnamon is also available in capsule form for those who might not like the taste if you are interested in the possibility of it lowering blood sugar.

Just be aware that sometimes the capsules can result in cinnamon flavored burps after you take them! This might not be a big deal for some but I found it not pleasant.

As for the glucose lowering claims, I don't think it did much of anything for me but like other things, everyone is different so it might work for you. If you want to try it, and you are not allergic to it, then go ahead. Do some before and after blood sugar testing using the same foods before and after adding cinnamon to see if you notice any difference.

The second tip is to use a tick of chewing gum as a way to keep food cravings at bay. Chewing the gum will signal your brain that you are eating and the saliva that the gum generates will help as well. If you get a craving pop a stick of gum in your mouth and chew away until the craving leaves.

If you do decide to chew gum make sure it is sugar free or sugarless gum so you are not adding carbs to your diet by chewing the gum. Also, use moderation. A few sticks of gum is fine. Chewing 10 packs a day is not.

Create a More

Active Lifestyle

Though no one really like to hear this, creating a more active lifestyle is a great thing for almost everyone. But if you are a diabetic, an active lifestyle is even more important. This is because exercise and adding more activity helps in several ways and not just in weight loss.

Losing weight is a goal for most overweight diabetics because carrying less weight also tends to reduce blood sugar levels as well. Losing 10% of your body weight can have a dramatic effect on lowering your A1c levels. But you don't have to lose the 10% to start seeing benefits.

ANY weight loss means your body has to work less to accomplish the same results. Less weight means you heart has to work less to pump blood through all your veins and arteries and that can reduce high blood pressure. Weight loss helps the body process sugar more efficiently as well which is why your A1c is reduced as you lose weight.

While dieting and watching what you eat can help you lose weight, exercise is also required to improve the weight loss process and to help the body build muscle. But some people hate to exercise and are not likely to become "gym rats" overnight. Nor do they have to be.

But adding more exercise into your lifestyle does not mean sweating it out in the gym or health club. Sometimes just adding more activity into your lifestyle may be all that is required. In some cases, this might be the only way to lose weight and get in better shape safely.

Try and identify easy ways that you can integrate more activity into your lifestyle. For example, where do you drive to that is so close you might walk to it?

Maybe instead of driving to the bank you might walk there. Or walk to the library or other location. This way you build exercise into your everyday routine.

Walking is a great way to add activity that is not too intense or potentially harmful. Many people try to exercise too hard or intensely at first and then hurt themselves or get discouraged. But almost everyone can walk so this might be a great way to start adding a little bit of activity.

Why not go for a walk after breakfast or lunch every day. You don't have to walk for miles and miles in order to see benefits. Aim for 30 minutes to start or whatever you are capable of. Maybe you start with just a walk around the block and go from there. Maybe you walk around the block once for a week and then try walking around it twice, then three times until you find your limit.

Even doing little things like parking further away from the store and walking those extra 50 steps can add up at the end of the week. In bad weather go out and walk the mall and window shop. Or just walk around the inside of the house for 15 to 20 minutes a few times a day.

Exercise will also help us build lean muscle and reduce fat content. If you have the ability, either get a scale that tests your BMI (Body Mass Index) or have your doctor show you how to calculate it for yourself. Your BMI is an indication on how fit your overall body is compared to fat and lean muscle content.

More lean muscle and less fat burn more calories and allow cells to process glucose more easily. It also helps reduce cholesterol levels which is extremely important because diabetics are more prone to coronary artery disease. Exercise and reduced cholesterol will lower your chances of developing heart disease in addition to all the other benefits.

It is not our goal to become a ripped person bulging with muscles. But exercise helps us look and feel better and helps our body better cope with glucose levels and fight diseases. There is no way that anyone cannot find some easy ways to add just a little bit of activity into their lifestyle.

Start small and go from there. It is not who gets the most exercise in the shortest amount of time who wins.

It is the person who finds small ways to make a long lasting change that comes out the winner. There is no reason why that winner cannot be you!

Lose a Bit of Weight

We just talked about adding some exercise into our lifestyle so we can look and feel better and help our bodies process sugars more efficiently. Weight loss is something that most of us have attempted at least once or twice in our lives but it now takes on a whole other significance.

Weight loss is important because the harder the body has to work in order to feed all its cells and organs, the more stress is placed on the parts of the body charged with doing those things. That means the heart has to work harder to push the blood through more veins and capillaries and the pancreas has to work harder to produce more insulin.

In diabetics, we usually have cells that are resistant to process glucose.

So we require more insulin in order to get the sugars into the cells where they are needed. This is why sugar levels in the blood rise sometimes uncontrollably. Anything we can due to lower the cells ability to process glucose will help us control our blood sugar.

Weight loss and exercise help us do that. And a lot more as well.

Weight loss is good for your entire body. The reduced weight eases the burden and stress of your hip joints and other weight bearing joints such as the knees. It promotes strength and reduces weakness. Assuming you are not already too thin, there is almost always a benefit in losing a few pounds.

But the question as a diabetic is how to safely go about losing that weight. Diets can be problematic because not only do you have to concern yourself with reducing calories, you also have to reduce those calories while maintaining the proper amount of carbohydrate while still giving your body the nourishment it needs to stay healthy and protect your body against other problems and diseases.

The answer usually lies with doing things in moderation. That means taking it slow and gradually so you can reach your goal without harming yourself or your body in the process. You also want to go about things in such a way that you will be able to sustain your efforts and not burn yourself out in the process.

Here are a few things to think about when it comes to weight loss:

Develop a Plan

Every weight loss effort should be done with a plan in place. That means knowing what you want to do and how to best go about achieving the desired results. You must be honest with yourself when designing your plan. Your plan should be designed well within your abilities so the effort is a long and sustained one. It is not smart to design a plan that will push you to the limits and cause you to just give up because you are asking too much of yourself.

Take it Slow

Whether you have to lose 10 pounds or 100 pounds, you cannot do it over night. Healthy weight loss takes time and sustained weight loss requires a change in your lifestyle that must be gradual and effective in order to remain in place. So it is far better to be slow and steady than to take it fast and crash and burn.

Depending on your particular situation, you should lose no more than two pounds a week and sometimes that might even be too much. Work with your doctor to come up with a weight loss schedule that is healthy and achievable. If that means you lose 2 pounds a week, then 2 pounds it is. If your doctor says one pound, then one pound is what you should do.

It is far better to lose one pound a week for 20 weeks than to lose 5 pounds the first week but give up because you cannot sustain the effort. Remember, that if you walk a half mile a day at the end of each month you have walked 15 miles. If you try to walk 2 miles and give up after 3 days you would have only walked 6!!!

Make it Healthy

Your body needs time to adjust to changes in diet and exercise. If your diet is too extreme your body will not get the nutrition it needs to do everything it needs to heal itself and protect itself against diseases and damage.

If you try to do too much exercise all at once you can damage muscles and bones and cause all kinds of health problems from strained muscles to fractures and back problems.

Also, take a look in the mirror and realize that when you are 40 you can't necessarily do the same things you could when you were 20. Even if you can still do them that doesn't mean that you should. While it is perfectly fine to push yourself a bit when you exercise, don't expect more from your body that it can safely deliver.

Moderate Exercise

As we stated when talking about weight loss, exercise should be moderated so we can safely do what we are trying to do without having to expend too much effort or have troubles after we are done.

If the sacrifice is too great, or if we are disappointed with our level of success, then we become unmotivated and we stop.

We should concentrate instead of exercising for longer periods of time instead of intensity. Granted we need a certain level of intensity to get the heart rate up but that doesn't mean trying to run the 3 minute mile or run the next marathon.

Start walking first and gradually increase the pace. Then mix walking and running doing alternating periods of each. Pick a time frame that works for you. At first you will walk more than run but that may change as you get into better shape. Then again, it might not.

Experts state that to get benefit from cardio exercise you should exercise for 30 minutes or more 5 days a week. Of course you could do more if you feel like it and your doctors agree, but 30 minutes should be the minimum of what you strive for. If you can't do 30 minutes at first then work up to it.

Work with your doctor to find the best exercise program for you. Some people might benefit from hiring a personal trainer at a local gym to design a workout plan that takes into consideration your personal physical condition and age. While this costs money, it will give you a healthy way to exercise. You might consider just a session or two so that you get the plan and then follow that plan on your own. Whatever works for you is best.

Keep Yourself Hydrated

Everyone needs to keep hydrated throughout the day and for diabetics this is even more important. Diabetics are more prone to kidney disease and dehydration can cause problems in the kidneys including the formation of kidney stones and other issues. Anyone who has ever had a kidney stone will tell you they are no fun at all so drink plenty of water.

Carry a water bottle with you when you exercise. If you wait until you are thirsty that is too late. You are already starting to dehydrate. Take frequent sips of water throughout your walk, run or workout.

Drink a glass of water before your workout and several glasses afterwards as your body heals and recovers from your exercise.

Some people limit water because water adds weight and they are trying to lose weight. But excess water is flushed from the body as urine so it doesn't accumulate like extra calories. While water might make you weight a pound more today it will be back to normal tomorrow when you become properly hydrated.

Check Your Sugar!

Exercise has a direct effect on blood sugar so the need to test before, sometimes during and after exercise is important. This will help you avoid low blood sugar episodes and other problems.

Check your blood sugar before you exercise, especially in the beginning so you can get an idea of how your body responds to exercise. In the beginning it might also be a good idea to test in the middle of the workout as well to see how exercise is being tolerated.

Then, test at the end of the workout to see where your sugars are then as well. After you have worked out for a while you usually will have a pretty good idea of what you can and can't do but at the beginning, this is a learning phase requiring testing.

Exercise has a side benefit of lowering blood sugar. This can continue for hours after you stop exercising which is a good thing as far as blood sugar control is concerned. But this also means if your sugars were controlled before you started exercising the new exercise might lower it further and result in low sugar episodes. These are not healthy and you should plan on avoiding them as much as possible.

Low sugars will make you feel weak, sweaty and just overall bad. The first time you might not realize this is a low sugar episode but if it is cold and you are sweating profusely, or if your legs are feeling weak or strange, check your sugars to make sure they are at normal levels. For some people, carrying a small amount of carbs with them on their run or walk might be a good idea.

A piece or two of hard candy, a small sugary drink or a glucose tablet should do the trick. Do NOT overdo it or you will find your blood sugars shooting way up after being so low. Take a bit of carbohydrate and retest in 15-20 minutes. You should start to feel better and stop sweating as your glucose levels begin to stabilize.

Have Medical Supervision

Before you start on your exercise or weight loss plan, have a talk with your doctor to make sure it is medically acceptable for you to do so. Some of us might have other conditions that prohibit certain types of exercise or restrict the amount of intensity of exercise.

Your goals should be health first and everything else second. Don't convince yourself that you can or should do more than what your doctor tells you. They have a reason for their instruction and even though we might not understand that reason, we should follow it.

If you have any questions, or if you disagree with the doctor, discuss it with them and never just take things into your own hands and do more than what you are supposed to do.

Track Your Progress

So much of exercise revolves around motivation. You need to be motivated to start doing something and once you have started, you need motivation to keep it up in order to get continued benefits. Once motivation ceases our chances of stopping are increased greatly.

One great way to keep motivated is to track your progress. Write down what you are doing and for how long. As you get in better physical condition you will see that you are walking further, running faster, lifting heavier weights or even seeing another notch on your belt. Whatever it might be, knowing and seeing your progress will help you keep up the effort.

For diabetics, you should track your sugar levels, weight loss and A1c levels as you exercise.

As you see your sugars decrease, that should motivate you. When you get the next A1c test results and see that they have gone down a half point, that should motivate yourself as well.

Also, though this might be hard to actually measure, try and realize if you feel better and look better. If you do this is a form of positive reinforcement that will help keep you motivated and engaged for longer periods of time.

Most people need to see and realize benefits of doing something that might not always be enjoyable or convenient. But the next time we might feel like sitting down and watching television instead of going out on a 30 minute run or walk, the positive results, and the motivation they bring with them, will help us get up and go out for that walk or run.

Use a Pedometer

or Exercise Band

It seems that we are in the middle of a fitness craze with all kinds of aids and devices to help us lose weight and feel better. While some of these devices might seem a bit weird or crazy, there are a few that make perfect sense when it comes to exercise, weight loss and controlling blood sugar. Two of these devices are pedometers and fitness bands. I have used both and I find both of them useful but for different reasons.

Pedometers are good for people who like to walk and for an indication of overall activity during the course of a normal or regular day.

The suggested fitness goal for a person wearing a pedometer is usually 10,000 steps a day. Depending on the length of your legs, that represents somewhere between 4 and 5 miles.

It is not all that easy to reach 10,000 during a normal day without doing some kind of formal or dedicating walking so the 10,000 level is good for just that reason. If you have a job where you sit behind a desk all day you might come home with less than 3,000-4,000 steps! If that is the case then you will need to add a walk before work, during lunch or after work to get up to the 10,000 step level.

The pedometer will give you an indication of just how active or sedentary you were during the day. It can give you a much needed kick in the pants to get you moving and it also can motivate you to do more and hit a new high. Feel free to set your own goal according to your schedule and availability. The more steps you make the more exercise you get!

Fitness bands are a more recent addition and they can help in pretty much the same way plus a few other ways.

Most of them will count steps like a pedometer but they will also track something called a "fuel unit" or similar name which takes other things other than steps in consideration.

The problem with pedometers is that they only count steps. So if I walk slowly for long enough I can still get my 10,000 in the course of the day without really getting much exercise or getting my heart rate up at all. With an exercise or fitness band, it will monitor speed, acceleration and depending on the particular band, other things well.

So you will earn more fuel points for running or jogging 10,000 steps than you would if you slowly walked those same 10,000 steps. This is a far more accurate indication of the amount of exercise you get throughout the day than just counting steps.

It is not possible to go into more detail when it comes to fitness or exercise bands because they are all different.

But regardless of which band you purchase or whether you use a band or a pedometer, the whole idea is to understand how active you are during the day and use the devices to see how you can get more activity in your life without sacrifice.

There is the issue of cost to be concerned about when deciding which is right for you. Pedometers can be purchased for as low as $10 and they can get more expensive as you add features and accuracy. Fitness bands, on the other hand, can cost several hundred dollars with the low end around $100. That might be a bit more than many of you want to spend and there is no law that says you must own either of these devices.

Both devices go a long way in motivating you to become more active and to give you an overall indication of how active you are during any given day. With this information in hand you can decide how much additional activity or exercise you need to add to your daily routine.

But the hard and honest truth is that neither of these devices are going to cause you to lose weight or lower your blood sugar if you don't use them and track the information they provide. The information itself will be meaningless if you don't use it. Buying a fitness or exercise band and not using it is much like joining a gym and never going!

Regardless of which device you won I suggest that you track your results by writing down your data every day so you can look back and see how much you exercised or moved every day of the week or month. Writing the data down will help you discover trends that may help you lose more weight and become more active.

Depending on the job you have, you might find yourself more or less active on weekdays than you are during the weekends. So while you get enough steps or exercise commuting to and from work and during work throughout the week, you might have to add a walk or two during the weekends to round things out.

Tracking data is also useful so that you can see your progress over time.

For example you might notice you averaged 10,000 steps a day last month but over 11,000 steps a day this month. This is because you are in better shape or are used to walking and are increasing your distance because you want to or like to.

You might also want to write down your blood sugar readings as well so you can see if there is any relationship or correlation between your exercise and blood sugar. Noticing this might help you get more motivated and change your behavior to get better and more efficient results.

So while neither of these devices will cause you to lose weight by itself, both of them will make it easier to identify ways of becoming more active and adding activity into your lifestyle. Both will also indicate when you have had a more active or less active day and give you the opportunity to add exercise or steps as necessary to help you remain on goal.

Leave the Car Home!

One easy way to lower your blood sugar is by adding activity into your lifestyle and a great way of doing that is to leave the car at home and walk to more place that you need to go. That means more steps and more activity and lower blood sugars.

But even if you have to take the car you can still add activity in your daily routine. Unless it is raining or really, really cold, why not park at the outer edge of the parking lot as far away from the entrance as possible? This will make you walk more just to get into the store. You can easily add 500 steps of more to your totals just by doing this little trick.

If someplace is close by and you don't have to carry heavy or bulky objects to or from the place then why not walk?

Once you are where you need to go, why not walk around a little bit inside the store instead of just going right to what you need and then right back out after you're done?

Not only will you get more exercise but you will save money on gas and add life to your vehicle as well. Just don't try and walk too far especially in the beginning. Pick somewhere close by and walk instead of drive. The more often you do this the more exercise you will get.

Monitor Blood Pressure

If you are a diabetic, you need to know your blood pressure to make sure it isn't too high. Diabetics are more prone to heart disease and other cardiac problems because of the added glucose present in our blood. High blood pressure will make a diabetic an even higher risk for these problems.

There are several ways to test your blood pressure.

Your doctor will take your blood pressure during every office visit and yearly physical. If they don't tell you what your pressure is, ask them. Just being told it is normal is not enough. Ask for the numbers.

You should know that blood pressure readings taken in the doctor's office are often higher because people are nervous or stressed when they go to see the doctor. So if they are a bit high it might not be a problem.

You can also test your blood pressure at one of the free machines located in most pharmacies. You place your arm in the hole, press a button and wait for the test to end. Your readings will be shown to you on the screen. One word of caution when it comes to these machine. Their accuracy might not be the best because they are used so much and sometimes abused by other people. If you get a high reading that is higher than what you are used to, you might want to see your doctor to have your pressure checked professionally.

One of the easiest, and sometimes best, ways to check your blood pressure is by purchasing a home blood pressure monitor. They are not expensive and when you have one you can easily check your pressure any time you want. You can check it in the morning, before bed, when you are feeling well and when you are feeling poorly.

Another good thing a home pressure monitor can do is allow you to see how your blood pressure changes when you are stressed or agitated for whatever reason. Sometimes stress will make your pressure go higher and sometimes this might be a concern.

Owning a blood pressure home kit will allow you to catch any potential blood pressure issues very early and allow them to be addressed before they can cause problems. This is very important because high blood pressure is called the "silent killer" because it sometimes has no symptoms whatsoever. In that regard high blood pressure is like high blood sugar levels. You can have them and never know it.

Have your blood pressure tested professionally at least once a year or at every doctors visit. Compare those readings with the ones you get at home to make sure your home device is still accurate and functioning properly. If you notice your blood pressure increasing over time, bring it to the attention of your doctor.

Factors that can make your blood pressure go higher are excessive weight, stress, exercise, sickness, fear, or high salt intake. If you should start getting higher readings than normal think back to see if any or all of these triggers became present in your life recently.

Monitor Cholesterol

Diabetics should also have their cholesterol checked on a regular basis and this is usually more than once a year. High cholesterol is an even bigger problem for those people with diabetes. Since high cholesterol is one of the risk factors for coronary artery disease, we need to keep a close eye on our cholesterol levels.

Though the suggested guidelines change over the years, usually cholesterol levels should be below 180 for non-diabetics and under 100 for diabetics. The lower levels are suggested for diabetics because they are at much higher risk for coronary artery disease and heart attacks.

Your endocrinologist will usually test for cholesterol as part of a basic metabolic panel blood test.

This is the test that also includes your A1c test as well as other basic blood tests. I have mine tested 3-4 times a year and you will probably get yours tested about the same number of times as well.

If cholesterol is an issue for you then it would be a good idea to consult a nutritionist or check with your doctor for suggestions on how to lower your cholesterol naturally. For those with higher cholesterol that is too high for natural control, then perhaps your doctor will prescribe a cholesterol lowering medication.

Many diabetics are on some form of cholesterol lowering drug because of the tighter standards for diabetics. So don't be afraid or worried if your doctor suggests a cholesterol drug. It doesn't necessarily mean you have a problem. It might mean you just want to prevent a problem from occurring.

Reduce Stress

Most people are aware that stress is not good for you. Stress can raise blood pressure and also raise blood sugars as well. Because of this, we should take steps to lower or reduce the amount of stress in our lives. Sometimes this is easier said than done but we should all try.

Stress places a strain on your entire body. It is just not blood pressure or blood sugar that is effected by stress. Stress effects our minds and brains and emotions as well. It just makes our bodies work harder to accomplish routine or everyday tasks.

There are several ways to reduce stress and some might be more effective for you than others. Naturally, removing the source of the stress is the best approach but that is often not an option. It is just not possible to remove all stress.

But sometimes we can do a few things to make stressful situation easier to handle.

First, try not to worry or get upset over things that are out of your control. You cannot control the weather, the actions of others and many other things that go on around us. For us to think we can influence or control these things is just not a rational response. So the best way for us to deal with this type of stress is to just "let go" of the situation and do our best to make the outcome as positive as possible.

Second, when we are feeling stressed, sometimes taking a few minutes to regain control will work wonders. We can take a moment to calm down, think things through and decide how to best proceed. Sometimes when we feel overwhelmed just thinking about it and sorting things out is enough to see that things aren't really all that bad.

Third, when you are feeling stressed or tense, take several deep breaths. Breathe in slowly and let the air out slowly. This will have a calming effect on your body, reduce heart rate and help you bring things back into control.

Fourth, and sometimes a real benefit to diabetics, find someone to talk to about the stress in your life. This might be a counselor or therapist or social worker. Sometimes when people are first diagnosed with diabetes they feel overwhelmed and afraid because they have a disease they know little about. Having someone to talk to and be reassured by can make all the difference in the world. This might not be the answer for some people but it might help a few people as well.

Exercise is also known to be a great stress reliever as well. Exercise will reduce frustrations, melt away stress, and give you a release for anger and other feelings. Plus, it will help you lower your blood sugar which stress can raise.

If you feel that stress is a big part of your live talk to your doctors about this. They can help point you in the right direction so that you can help deal with stress more effectively in the future. We all have a certain amount of stress in our lives. Some of us just know how to deal with it better.

Check Your Feet

Every Day

Your doctor probably talked to you about this but because this is so important, we wanted to make sure we covered it here as well. What I am referring to is the need to check your feet every day to make sure they are in good condition.

Diabetics are more prone to infections and other diseases that can occur and enter the body through cuts or cracks in the skin. Our feet are primary places for this to happen. Plus, because our feet are encased on shoes all day long the environment is dark and damp and that is a perfect breeding ground for infections and fungus.

We should check our feet every day for breaks in the skin, ingrown toenails, callouses and other problems such as blisters, rashes, and fungus. The presence of any of these conditions means that we need to take action sooner rather than later before more serious problems occur.

Trim toenails with smooth edges so they don't puncture the skin. Do not try and trim nails too far down. You do not want to expose the soft skin normally protected by the nail or cut the skin while trimming the nail. Cut the nail but leave a little bit exposed underneath to protect the skins under the nail.

Check the bottom of the feet for blisters and callouses and address any issues you may find. If blisters have "popped" then apply an ointment to keep them from getting infected. If it is possible to use a Band-Aid or pad to protect the skin during the healing process that is good as well.

Apply foot cream to soften callouses or use an abrasive pad or other method designed to remove callouses to soften the skin.

When callouses are allowed to get thick they can result in cracking of the skin which is not only painful, the cracks can allow bacteria and fungus into the body and we need to avoid that.

As far as footwear and socks are concerned, try and wear shoes that allow the foot to breathe. Leather is a better material than plastic. Cheap shoes often do not breathe very well and the results is the feet get very moist. This is the perfect environment for fungus to grow.

Shoes should also fit well and should not be too tight or too loose. When shoes are too tight they can damage feet and impede the circulation of blood. When they are too loose, the move around excessively and this can result in blisters especially at the back of the foot. Get fitting properly for your shoes.

If you wear socks, try and get good quality socks that can wick away moisture while being soft and thick enough to provide cushioning for the feet. This is important if you do a lot of walking, running or jogging. Every step you take places pressure on the bottoms of your feet and the combination of socks and footwear provide protection for your feet.

There are special running shoes available that help provide the protection and support your feet need when walking or running. They are also light weight so this takes a little bit of the pressure off the feet as well. Whatever design you choose make sure your shoes provide the proper support and that they are well ventilated so your feet can breathe.

If you should encounter any issues while examining your feet, take care of them as soon as possible. Do not think the problems will go away by themselves. Trim nails often and properly and treat any cracks or callouses immediately. If you should encounter a rash or fungus, or anything that looks out of the ordinary, see your doctor as soon as possible. You do not want a little problem to become a big problem.

See an Eye Doctor

at Least Once a Year

Diabetics should have their eyes examined once a year. More often if your doctor recommends. This is because diabetics are more prone to certain eye problems because the higher glucose levels can cause problems within the eye.

The eye is full of tiny, tiny blood vessels that can become damaged when glucose levels are high for extended periods of time. This is a disease called retinopathy. People with retinopathy can lose part or all of their vision if the disease is allowed to progress.

Fortunately, there are medications designed to slow down the process and that, along with proper blood sugar control can help prevent this kind of problem.

But in order to treat the problem you need to become aware of it. Since retinopathy may have no symptoms, or very gradual ones, an eye exam is needed to look at the back of the eye for damage.

This is more than your standard eye exam that you get when you need glasses. This is a full exam done by a doctor not a clerk behind a counter. If you already have an eye doctor that you see every year, that's great. If you don't have one, ask your doctor or endocrinologist to recommend one for you.

Follow your doctor's recommendation as far as how often you should get your eyes checked. As already stated, usually this is once a year but if you have eye problems already, or if you have been diagnosed already with retinopathy, then you might have to do more often.

Do not take this lightly as we only have one pair of eyes and once we lose our sight life becomes very different. The things you and I take for granted are very much missed by people who have lost their sight. So make the time and pay the co-pay for an eye doctor visit to protect your eyesight.

Stop Smoking

No one should smoke, period. There is just too much evidence and too many studies showing the horrible and life-changing damage tobacco products can do to you for anyone to continue smoking. Contrary to what many people say, smoking isn't cool or the popular thing anymore. So if you smoke stop and if you haven't started yet, don't start.

Diabetics have problems when their bodies are under stress and tobacco products cause blood vessels to change, interfere with normal lung function and cause diseases that most healthy people with normal immune systems have a hard time fighting.

Diabetics are more sensitive to infection and other things that make our bodies work harder to perform normal body functions.

When the body has to work harder blood sugars often rise. When a diabetic gets an infection or a disease, treatment becomes more difficult because not only do we have to fight the disease, we have to concern ourselves with blood sugar levels as well. This might render certain treatments unavailable for some patients.

Not smoking is just another way we can help our bodies stay healthier longer and help us keep our sugars under control. Anything we can do that allows the body to do what it needs to easier and faster is a good thing for diabetics. So again, if you are currently smoking, please stop. And if you are not a smoker now, please don't become one.

Also, if you are a smoker in the same house as a diabetic, quit for their sake if you won't quit for yours. Second hand smoke has been shown to be very deadly to those who live around smokers. So please look around you and if you see other people, especially children and grandchildren, give them a special gift by not smoking. You will help stay in their lives longer and help them live longer and healthier lives at the same time.

This isn't a diabetic vs. non-diabetic issue. It is a healthy vs. unhealthy lifestyle issue.

If you are a smoker and wish to quit, there are many products available to help you quit without experiencing the full effects of withdrawal. But before you use any of these products talk to your doctor or endocrinologist to make sure these products are safe for diabetics and that they will not make your sugars go up from their use. Your doctor may also prescribe some more powerful medication designed to make it even easier for you.

There is no better time to start than right now. Not tomorrow or next month but right now. The only thing worse than a patient with lung cancer is a diabetic with lung cancer.

Get Flu Shots

Every Year

This is a quick and easy one. Check with your doctor about getting a flu shot every year. If there is no medical reason why you shouldn't or can't get a flu shot, then get one. Diabetics have a tougher time fighting disease and the flu is no different.

When a diabetic gets a cold or the flu or any kind of infection, the body has to work harder to fight off the infection. That places the body in stress and this raises blood sugars. So it makes sense to do whatever you can to minimize your chances of getting the flu.

Make sure you dress warmly and try and distance yourself from those you know are sick. This can be difficult in the office or when you are caring for a sick family member but at other times, try and distance yourself from others who look like they are sick or have a cold.

The flu is a miserable disease that can knock you out for a week or more. So get the flu shot and live a healthy lifestyle and you should have a good chance of escaping the flu.

Oh, no!

That Was 26 Ways
Already!

We Still Have
More to Share!

How About Some
"Bonus Content"?

Just Turn the Page!

Replace Sugary Drinks

with Tea or Water

Though many of us know this, some of us ingest thousands of calories each and every week by drinking sugary and calorie laden beverages with our meals and snacks and sometimes just to quench our thirst. While these drinks do nothing for us other than help us gain weight and feel bloated, they also have a profound effect on our blood sugar levels!

Depending on your drink of choice, sodas can have 50 or more grams of carbohydrates in a single can! That is more than many people consume in an entire meal! 50 grams of carbs is enough to make our blood sugars rise even if we don't eat a single thing with that drink!

When you add the carbs in a regular meal, even a healthy meal, the sugars just skyrocket!

What is even worse, those 50 grams of carbohydrate and sugar is just for one little 12 ounce can! If you have a 20 ounce bottle that could mean 80 or more grams and if you go to a fast food place and get one of their super large mega gulp gigunda size drinks you might be ingesting hundreds of grams of carbohydrates just from your drink!

Here is an example that might put things into perspective:

Early after my diagnosis I went to a fast food place and bought a roast beef sandwich and a large soft drink. I skipped the fries because fries are high in carbs and, well, they are fried which is not good for you either. Back then my "resting sugars" were about 110 to 120. Two hours after I ate I tested my sugars to make sure they were OK and to my shock I found they were over 300!!!

I did some research and found out the huge amounts of carbs in the giant drink and knew why my sugars were so high.

So I made a promise never to subject my body to that much soda again. Changes were in order and I knew I had to make them. Sometimes we need an experience like that to set us straight!

In addition to the carb levels, the calories alone are good reasons to stop consuming these beverages. A single can of soda can have 150 calories in it. So with just one can per day, you are consuming an additional 1,000 calories a week or 52,000 calories a year! With one pound equal to approx. 3,500 calories, one can of soda per day can add up to roughly 14-15 pounds of extra weight per year!!!

Or, it means that you have to exercise that much more to just stay at your own weight at the end of every week. See how long you have to walk on a treadmill to burn off those 150 calories in a single can of soda. That might make you reconsider what you should be drinking with meals and snacks.

On a nutrition standpoint, they do not call sodas and other sugary drinks "empty calories" for nothing. Other than an energy boost from the sugars these beverages offer nothing positive or good for your body.

They taste good and that's about it. Other than taste, they are no good for you and almost everyone can find a different beverage that they find tastes good as well.

Some people substitute diet drinks for the sugary versions and that is good when it comes to carbs but diet sodas have artificial sweeteners and those have been known to cause problems of their own and sometimes they can effect blood glucose as well.

Carbonated drinks and certain other drinks also have a lot of salt or sodium in them and that not only causes you to gain "water weight" but it also helps you feel thirstier faster so you want to drink more and more! Plus, there are artificial flavors, coloring, preservatives and lord knows what else in them. So while diet beverages are better than regular ones, there are better choices.

Water is the best overall choice because it is just, well, water. It hydrates us, gives our bodies what they need to properly nourish our cells and have none of the salt and other garbage processed beverages have.

You can drink as much water as you want as long as you are within reach of the rest room!

If you don't like drinking water, try unsweetened beverages like iced tea and seltzer. But watch the other ingredients in these beverages to make sure they are what they say they are. Just because something says it is low sugar or low sodium does not mean it has NO sodium or NO sugar. Low can be a relative term so read and compare nutrition labels.

Try and drinks teas and low calorie beverages whenever you can't have water or don't want to have water. While it is OK to have a soda or other higher calorie beverage as a treat once in a while, it is not a good thing to make them a frequent or permanent part of your everyday diet. All restaurants serve water and every fast food restaurant will give you water if you ask for it. Everyone MUST drink a certain amount of water each day to keep themselves properly hydrated. Water is good for you and is a healthy beverage.

Water helps your kidneys flush waste and toxins from your body and drinking plenty of water helps prevent kidney stones.

Other beverages actually might help form stones so why take the chance? Drink water as often as possible and help protect your body and help it flush itself free of toxins and other substances. Water also helps fight constipation as well.

So let's all just start drinking more and more water, OK?

Vinegar May Reduce

Glucose Surge

Talk to your doctor regarding adding a little bit of vinegar to your diet. Studies have shown that people who consume a bit of vinegar in or with their meals have lower and more slowly rising blood glucose levels.

While no one is really sure why this happens, it might be worth a try to see if it works for you. Be sure to test your blood sugar before and after adding vinegar using the same foods to see if it really does help you.

But be careful not to ingest too much vinegar because too much is not always better. Stick to recommended levels. Some studies show that ingesting two teaspoons of vinegar before meals does help with glucose levels. Try adding roughly two teaspoons of vinegar to your meals to start.

As with any food, you should make sure your body can handle the food and that you are not allergic to anything or have any disease or medical condition that might be effected by adding vinegar to your diet. If you are already using vinegar in your foods this should not be an issue but you should check with your doctor first.

Naturally, if you are allergic or have any digestive reaction when you consume vinegar you should not add vinegar to your diet.

Never Adjust Meds Without Doctors Approval

The medications that our doctors prescribe us are designed to help keep our blood glucose levels stable and help us manage the rest of the aspects of diabetes. This can include cholesterol, blood pressure, eye and kidney problems and anything else that might be involved.

These medications sometimes work independently and some work in conjunction with other medications. But even the medications that work independently can sometimes interact with other medications.

That is why it is very important to keep taking your meds as directed. Take the dosage that is prescribed and if you should miss a dose accidently, follow the directions for that medication. Do not just double up on the next dose or take a random action.

When it comes to medication do not increase or decrease the dosage unless directed by your physician. If your sugars are high do not take more medication. If they are low do not take less. Take the recommended dosage only. If you have reservations or fear about continuing a medication, talk to your doctor first.

The same applies to stopping medications for any reason. If a medication has an unpleasant side effect and you want to stop taking that medication, do not just stop. Let your doctor know. Some medications can be dangerous if stopped suddenly. Some medications need to be stopped gradually over time and on a specific schedule to avoid side effects and damage to the body.

Changing the dosage or stopping a medication might not have the effect you think it is going to have.

Only your doctor can tell you the safest way to get certain results. If a medication is bothering you perhaps there is a different but similar medication that can achieve the same results but without the unpleasant side effects. But only your doctor can tell you that.

Also, and this should be common sense, take only those medications prescribed for you. If you have a family member, friend or co-worker who has diabetes and they rave about their medications, do NOT take any of their medication. If you think this medication might be good for you then ask your doctor about it. Chances are if this medication was a really good fit for you they would have already had you on it. Trust your medical team and talk about your medications with them.

If you are seeing more than one doctor, for example a family doctor and an endocrinologist, make each doctor aware of any changes in medications prescribed by the other doctors in your medical team. This is important because any additional medications you are given might change the medications prescribed by another doctor.

Some medications do not work well together and some medications should not be taken at the same time. So your doctor might alter the time you take each medication or the dosage so everything works well together. But they can only do this when they are aware of everything you are taken.

For this reason, and to make sure you are on the proper medications, make it a part of every appointment to bring each doctor up to date on the medications you are currently taking. This would include new meds and meds you are no longer taking.

Everything works better when everyone involved is well informed.

Join a Support Group

Sometimes it's nice to have company when you are trying to accomplish something that is a bit overwhelming or when you are not sure how to best go about it. Sometimes you might even think that your problem or troubles are unique to you and that there is no one who can possibly help you let alone understand what you are going through.

In other words, sometimes we feel all alone out there with a disease that initially frightens us a bit and leaves us wondering what to do first and how to get where we need to go in controlling things. For many people, a diabetes support group is the perfect solution for a lot of people who want help and need help but either don't know where to find it or can't afford it.

Check with your doctor or endocrinologist to find a program in your area. You might also try the local hospital. Many hospitals have their own diabetes care and support groups and these are either free or very low cost. You can also try the various organizations dedicated to the fight against diabetes as well.

Groups will not only supply support but also knowledge on how to deal with the side effects of the disease and how to lower blood sugar. They will provide nutritional counselling or show you where to find it and they might even recommend a new doctor if you need to find one.

Sometimes feeling alone is just as bad as the disease itself. There is no reason today why anyone has to go through any disease all by themselves. If you want or need support, it is there for you.

All you need to do is look for it.

Brush, Floss, and

See a Dentist Regularly

Though you might not think about it much, your dental hygiene is important when it comes to managing your blood sugars. This is because poor dental hygiene can lead to infections, open gum sores, tooth decay and gum disease.

All of the above can play havoc with blood sugar levels. For example, a few years back my sugars rose suddenly by over 100 points and no one could figure out why. Then, I got a toothache and had to have root canal to clear out an infection within the tooth. After that procedure was done the sugars dropped back to normal! The high sugars were a warning that something was wrong and that was the infection that had just started!

See your dentist every 6 months and have an examination of your teeth and gums. Have your teeth cleaned to protect both your teeth and gums. This can not only make you feel better and be healthier but it can protect you against tooth loss as well.

As for daily care, be sure to brush after every meal. If you cannot brush them at least rinse food particles out of your mouth. Floss regularly also to get rid of food that is stuck between teeth. All of this will take you only minutes a day and can save you a lot of money on dental work as well as improving your overall oral health.

Get a Full Night's

Sleep Every Night

While everyone benefits from getting a full night's sleep, diabetics need their rest even more than non-diabetics. Sleep is the time where our body tries to recover from the day's events and rebuild and heal itself to prepare for the next day.

When we try to do too much and neglect our rest, several things happen. Our bodies don't get a chance to fully heal and therefore may not be ready for what happens the next damage. We might not have the strength or stamina we usually have and our ability to concentrate and react to certain things might be impaired as well.

Lack of proper rest and sleep places the body under additional stress and that tends to raise our blood sugar levels. Getting the proper amount of rest allows our body to function better the following day and to be more relaxed and healthy.

There is some debate on what constitutes a full night's sleep. The standard answer is that 8 hours of sleep is what most people should have. Now if we get 7 hours and 45 minutes of sleep that is close enough. But 4 or 5 hours is not enough for anyone. Every diabetic should develop a schedule where they get 8 hours of quality, uninterrupted sleep every night.

Uninterrupted sleep is one of the keys because 8 hours of continuous and uninterrupted sleep is not the same as grabbing 8 one hour naps over the course of the day.

Stay Away from Steroids

I know, I know, everyone should stay away from steroids! But the steroids I am referring to are not the same steroids that athletes and body builders use to give themselves huge muscles and power. The steroids I am referring to are medications that might be steroid based. The most common are anti-inflammatories.

A few years back I had problems with my shoulder. The doctor injected a steroid based medicine in my shoulder and it really did help. Most of the pain was gone and I had full use of the shoulder without pain or discomfort.

However, I also had blood sugar that never went below 280 for the next two weeks! All because of the steroid based medication!

If you go to any doctor and they want to give you steroid based medication, check with your endocrinologist before allowing the medication to be given or before you take any pills. The endocrinologist will either want to prescribe additional medications to help further lower your sugars or they may advise you not to take the medication.

The most common example would be to treat poison ivy. I had that as well and the injection caused by sugars to go into the high 200's as well. But it also got rid of the poison ivy!

The motto is, do not take any medication that contains steroids, including over the counter products, without talking to your doctor first. If, for some reason you must take a steroid based drug in an emergency, make your doctor aware of it as soon as possible so they can help minimize the glucose spiking.

Talk to Your Doctor

About Supplements

Go to any supermarket or drug store today and you will see shelves of all different kinds of vitamins and supplement all of which are available without a prescription. But just because you don't need a prescription does not mean that these products are safe for diabetics.

Anything that we ingest has the possibility of effecting our blood sugar either positively or negatively. Sometimes even food that we eat can interfere with the way our medicines work once they are in our bodies.

Grapefruit, for example, is said to interfere with certain cholesterol medications. Certain over the counter medications interfere with medicines that control how our blood will clot. Even certain vegetable might cause us problems without us becoming aware of this.

But when it comes to supplement, these can also impact how other medications operate in our bodies. Vitamins can interfere with medications as can weight loss supplements and body building supplements. So before you decide to take a vitamin or any kind of supplement run the idea past your doctor first to make sure what you want to take is compatible with your medicines and health.

Do not believe that just because something says "healthy" or "safe" or "Natural" means you can take it with confidence. All of those might very well be true but they can still impact our health. So read labels and instructions carefully on all your medications and supplements before taking them.

Create a Testing

Routine

Though some of you might think this should have been among some of the first tips, we thought we would save it for the near the end so that after reading all the tips we can go over how to best monitor your sugars and get accurate results so you can do the right things at the right time.

First of all, remember that when you go for blood work that your glucose and A1c test MUST always be done in the morning and before you have had anything to eat. This is called a FASTING test which means no food after midnight before the morning of the test.

If you do eat your morning sugars will be high and this will not allow your doctor to get as accurate overall picture of how your body is processing sugar. A fasting test will let the doctor see how your sugars are first thing in the morning after your body has digested and processed what was eaten the day before.

Another important reason is that sometimes blood sugars will actually go up in the middle of the night even though you are not eating anything at the time. So a fasting test will let the doctor see what your sugars are at the start of every day.

When it comes to daily testing, your doctor will give you directions on when to test and how many times per day. If you are a "new" diabetic with fairly well controlled glucose levels and a low A1c your doctor might only want you to test once a day. If your glucose levels and A1c are higher, or if you are sick, they might want you to test more often. Follow you doctor's testing schedule as closely as possible.

After meal testing should be done 2 hours after a meal.

This will give your body a chance to digest some of the meal and allow you to see how your body is processing the foods you eat and help you decide whether or not you should continue to eat those food and in those quantities. If you test earlier than two hours you will get higher reading largely due to fast acting carbs that were in your meal.

If you are testing just once a day, try to make it the same time every day so you can compare like results. Testing today at 9AM and tomorrow at 9PM is not a good testing schedule. It is hard to compare readings taken at different times of the day and make accurate decisions. Discuss the best times that you can test every day and develop a testing plan that you can keep.

You should also test whenever you feel that you might be experiencing a low sugar condition. This might be accompanied by heavy sweating, weakness in your extremities or other abnormal or strange feelings. The first time you get a low sugar episode you might not realize what is going on. After a few you will be able to recognize their onset.

When you have a low sugar episode test yourself to see how low you have gone so you know what you have to eat to bring your sugars back up to normal. Then, it is usually said that you should test about 15 minutes later to see if they have come up to where you want them to be. Don't eat too much to get out of a low sugar episode. When you eat too much you might get a large swing from very low to very high.

Test strips and needles are not inexpensive but most insurance covers at least part of the cost. Do not stop testing or reduce testing to save a few dollars. Knowing what you blood sugar is each day is a critical part of managing your blood glucose levels. After all, you cannot manage what you are not aware of.

Next we will learn how to track our testing results.

Keep a Testing

& Food Log

Anyone who has tried to lose weight and involved a weight loss program or nutritionist probably was told about the need to fill out a food journal. While, when you are a diabetic you should see the value in filling out not only a food journal but a testing journal as well. In fact, a history of your testing will probably be part of your endocrinologist you get your A1c and overall control into the desired level.

Food journals are books where you write down everything that you eat and when you ate it. Then, at the end of the day or week, you go back to see what you ate and what the results were. Did you gain or lose weight? Were your glucose levels good or higher than usual?

If everything was what you expected or wanted then you had a good indication of what you could eat the next week to get the same results. But if the results were bad, such as a weight gain or higher glucose levels at times, you could look back and identify what caused the problems.

You see, sometimes it is not the scheduled meals that do you in but the little nibbles and snacks you have all the other times. You know what I am talking about. The chips you munched on or the 3 or 4 candies you took as you walked past the candy dish or the cookie you took from the cookie jar 4 times yesterday.

All of those little things can add up at the end of the day or week. It might not be difficult to pick up an additional 1,000 calories and 50 grams of carbohydrate from all of those "little" snacks and munchies. But if you wrote them all down you could see what the results of eating all that stuff really were. Sometimes that is enough to change your bad habits.

A testing journal, on the other hand, is just a listing of the results you had when you tested yourself throughout the day or week.

Writing these things down will help you spot trends and problems at an early stage when it is easier to manage them.

You can look at your testing journal to see when your sugars were higher or lower and then go to your food journal to see what you were eating at that time. Over time you will get a pretty good idea of what causes your highs and lows and then you can adjust your diet accordingly. Journals are just one more tool that you can use to discover the real reasons behind what is going on with your diabetes and your weight.

Journals will point out the things you never realized were in play. Journals will enable you to connect testing results with actual food and activities (if you track those as well!) so you can see how your body responded to different things.

Information is knowledge and knowledge helps you make better decisions, eliminate or at least reduce guesswork, and make fewer mistakes and waste less time. All of these things will help you gain control of your blood sugar faster and easier.

Conclusion

Diabetes is a serious illness but fortunately it is an illness that we can have a significant impact on. Many people have lived normal lives with the disease by just making the right choices at the right time and doing the little things to help keep blood glucose levels in check.

There is a ton of information in this book and it is all focused on giving you the tools you need to get a handle on glucose control and allow you to keep your diabetes in check.

Not everything in this book will be relevant to you and that's ok. It just means there is less for you to do every day when it comes to controlling your blood sugar. But also keep in mind that things change over time and what you don't have to do today you very well may have to do tomorrow.

Blood sugar control is a work in progress. There will always be changes that need to be made and adjustments to diet and medications but that's OK as well. Our bodies change over time. As we get older things don't work as well as they used to and we need to help them out a little bit with medication and lifestyle adjustments.

We are not invincible but we are not helpless in this fight either. In fact, if you do what is need to be done we can kick diabetes side effects in the butt and lead normal and healthy lives.

It's all in the knowledge and the attitude. We have given you the knowledge. The attitude is up to you!